THE INVISIBLE STROKE

VERONICA WOODS

authorHOUSE

AuthorHouse™ UK
1663 Liberty Drive
Bloomington, IN 47403 USA
www.authorhouse.co.uk
Phone: 0800 047 8203 (Domestic TFN)
　　　+44 1908 723714 (International)

© 2019 Veronica Woods. All rights reserved.

No part of this book may be reproduced, stored in a retrieval system, or transmitted by any means without the written permission of the author.

Published by AuthorHouse 04/09/2020

ISBN: 978-1-7283-9611-8 (sc)
ISBN: 978-1-7283-5237-4 (hc)
ISBN: 978-1-7283-9610-1 (e)

Print information available on the last page.

Any people depicted in stock imagery provided by Getty Images are models, and such images are being used for illustrative purposes only.
Certain stock imagery © Getty Images.

This book is printed on acid-free paper.

Because of the dynamic nature of the Internet, any web addresses or links contained in this book may have changed since publication and may no longer be valid. The views expressed in this work are solely those of the author and do not necessarily reflect the views of the publisher, and the publisher hereby disclaims any responsibility for them.

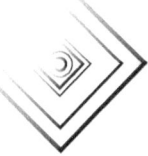

FOREWORD

Veronica Woods is a 46-year-old black British doctor. She graduated from Leicester Medical School in 1996. She is a very caring and resilient person. I admire her honesty and bravery in writing this book aimed at people who have an illness or disease that is not visible to the outside world. They suffer in silence.

Time and chances happen to us all. There are a lot of things that are happening around us. Some of these things we think we can control, but in the bigger picture, not everything is in our hands even though we are going through the motions. The strong and swift, the skilful and understanding, the slow and swift, the weak and strong, the unwise and wise—everything that happens to them may seem casual, but what we call chance is actually what has been ordered by God's divine providence. This time, chance has allowed and enabled Veronica Woods to tell the rest of the world her story of stroke, brain surgery, resilience, justice, personality changes, criminal conviction, and behavioural challenges.

This book is an eye-opener to the myriad of things that happen to stroke survivors. Most of the things covered here are not visible to the naked eye, but from Veronica Woods's point of view and experience, they are as real as they can get. Apart from being a stroke survivor, she has worked for twenty-two years for the National Health Service. She also writes about being an occupational health technician. Veronica writes about her battle with the large organisations to recognise her complex disorder and not to discriminate against her disability.

Veronica Woods left clinical practice immediately after her stroke as she was aware of the subtle changes in her cognition that may have affected her decision-making as a doctor.

Unfortunately, many health professionals did not understand her disease, which led to isolation, failed job opportunities, career loss, poor relationships with her family, and changed relationships with her friends. It therefore takes great commitment and passion in her career to accomplish the writing of this book while she is just months into recovery. Part of the reason why this book was written is because stroke is a misunderstood condition. Most people, including caregivers and general health practitioners, really do not know how to handle and treat stroke survivors in the early stages. Instead, survivors are subjected to a trial and error method of treatment just to get along and see what will work for them.

Stroke is indeed a complex phenomenon, but it has just gotten a little less complex. Dr Veronica Woods talks about being a doctor and a patient, including the fear of realising the effect of the disease also known as Takayasu's arteritis and pulseless disease. She talks honestly about her experience, and the hope is that stroke survivors, caregivers, general health practitioners, and the public will find this book important and helpful in demystifying stroke as well as finding the proper regiment or therapy to make life as normal as possible for every stroke survivor.

I would like to recognise Veronica Woods, the brains and inspiration behind this book. Her resilience and commitment to writing this book are proof that we can accomplish anything we put our minds to. I can never forget times when Veronica would have to be rushed to hospital while I was getting through the early stages of preparing this book. I thank God for giving her energy and health to see this book to completion.

This book would also have not been possible without Stephen Waititu Kamau, who co-authored, prepared, and organised the book.

Stephen Waititu Kamau is a Kenyan citizen aged 30 years. I consider myself a problem-solver and a computer geek. I was born in Kiambu County and went through the primary (Gakoe Primary School) and secondary (Mbugiti High School) part of the Kenyan education system in the same central region of Kenya. I was blessed with parents and guardians who valued education, and I love learning so I worked hard and smart to earn a bachelor of science degree at Egerton University, where I specialised in physics. It was during this stage of my life that I took up academic writing as a part-time occupation to support my family. As a graduate, I remain interested and passionate about learning, and as a millennial, computers are my tools of choice.

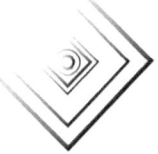

My Journal

By Veronica Woods

Early in 2012, I collapsed at a friend's house after work. It had been an ordinary day working as a GP. I had been looking forward to seeing my beautiful 4-year-old daughter and my loving husband that evening. There had been no warning: I was a keen runner, 36 years old, fit, and healthy. I was in the prime of my life.

My husband, also a GP, got the call, picked me up, and took me to the hospital, where the doctors performed a CT brain scan to surprise me with the diagnosis that would change my life forever.

The diagnosis was not good. I had suffered a brain haemorrhage, specifically a pontine haemorrhage with subarachnoid extension and internal carotid artery occlusion secondary to Takayasu arteritis disease.

Haemorrhages

A haemorrhage is what happens when a blood vessel like a vein or an artery weakens or bursts, letting blood into the surrounding tissue.

This means blood cannot get to where it is meant to and builds up where it shouldn't.

Pontine Haemorrhage and Subarachnoid Haemorrhage

When a haemorrhage happens in the brain, parts of the brain are starved of oxygen, causing them to be damaged or to die. The build-up of blood puts pressure on other parts of the brain, causing them to stop working properly or at all. This is why many people die or suffer brain damage from a haemorrhage in the brain.

Things Didn't Look Good

My prospects did not look good: most people don't survive a haemorrhage to the pons.

I was terrified. I couldn't walk or do anything by myself and was admitted to the local stroke unit for two weeks. I felt extremely vulnerable. I even called the doctor on call because I was so scared. The treatment I received at the unit was excellent, but I was not expecting to survive.

Explaining what was happening to my daughter was one of the most difficult parts. She was scared and didn't understand what was happening to me. My husband knew the chances of me dying and found it difficult to handle. He focused on keeping my daughter's life as normal as possible, and the distraction of selling our house kept him occupied.

The New 'Normal'

After two weeks, I was discharged from the hospital and given a panic alarm that would contact the emergency services if I pressed it. My life at home was completely different from how it had been before; I used to run, but now I could barely walk. I was dizzy and lightheaded and utterly terrified. Nothing felt normal. I didn't know if what I felt sometimes was the condition getting worse or just the new normal.

My family tried to continue with their lives around me. My husband went back to work, and my daughter went to school. My mum, dad, and sisters told me they were very scared, but they stayed strong. I don't think they knew how to respond to what was happening, but they supported me every inch of the way. I would sleep through the day and try to move as little as possible, worried I would collapse again. Anxiety and exhaustion filled my days as I waited for the results of more tests at the hospital.

Hopelessness

I couldn't see any hope. I thought my computer had crashed, and without it, the rest of me wouldn't survive. I thought I was broken. The woman my husband had married wasn't the woman I now was. The daughter I needed to be strong for needed me in ways I couldn't fulfil. I didn't want to leave them behind, and I prayed a lot for help and guidance. How could I live up to who I was? How could I work as a GP again? How could I run? What was life without these things?

Surgery and Hope

Four months after the initial haemorrhage, my stroke consultant referred me to a specialised hospital for further investigations. The results were shocking. My pre- and post-Acetazolamide SPECT scan and further MRI scanning, including BOLD reactivity, confirmed a bilateral reduction in cerebral vascular reserve that was worse on the left. My MRI scan showed scattered white areas in both my parietal and frontal regions consistent with ischaemic change.

The images were enough to meet the criteria for a superficial temporal artery-middle cerebral artery bypass operation. This would route a blood supply past the interrupted supply and connect the parts of my brain that had been starved of a proper blood supply.

This would route blood from the artery at the side of my face to the middle of my brain. I knew the chances of survival were low for this kind of operation, but I knew all surgery carries a risk, especially in the brain. It was very scary, but I felt so terrible I was prepared to do anything to feel better.

The surgeon was incredible. He was inspiring and reassured me a great deal. When I woke up from surgery, I immediately felt better. My vision had improved, my mood was lighter (not just from being alive), and I could see hope.

I thanked my surgeon again and again. I owe him everything. He is a miracle maker sent from God. I didn't know what would happen in my life or my family, but I knew I had to keep going for my little girl. The thought of her drove me on.

My Recovery Begins

It was a few days before I left hospital because I had a large hole in my skull that needed to start healing properly. The scar ran down the left side of my skull where the surgeon had to cut through skin and bone to get to my brain, sewing and stapling it shut afterwards. The whole side of my face had swelled up, but I was just happy to be alive and feeling better.

I received excellent care from the doctors and nurses both in and out of hospital, and the support they gave was invaluable. Recovering from brain surgery is confusing, scary, and painful, and the team around me, as well as my family, helped make it as good as it could be.

The ward was full of complex neurosurgical cases, including people going through tumour removal or recovering from brain damage. The brain is a very complex organ and can be changed so easily. Seeing other people in these conditions was reassuring because they were getting better and going home and scary because some of them had such severe damage.

The first few weeks were disorientating and full of worry. My head felt strange, like it wasn't mine, and it was very painful. We stayed in a flat near the hospital for a few days just in case something happened. I worried all the time. Had the sutures held? Would there be another bleed? Would I get my full functioning back?

As time passed, the consequences of the haemorrhage and the surgery were becoming clear. While I was recovering well, I wasn't the same person I had been. What had been easy before was now difficult. I felt a lot of neurological pain and my emotions were all over the place, but I had to keep going for my family.

One Month On

The brutal combination of healing, painkillers, and fatigue meant that the simple task of getting my daughter ready for school was so exhausting I would sleep for the rest of the day. Things were so difficult we hired a nanny, but my daughter was so attached to me she wouldn't accept one. It took a few tries before we got one she would tolerate. This was really difficult to accept. My husband and I used to do everything for the family, but now we needed extra help.

Throughout everything, I was supported by my GP, who continues to be wonderful. Now I could understand what my patients had been going through. I couldn't do much more than watch *The Real Housewives of New York City* during the day, and walking and eating were difficult but getting better. I could navigate around the home at least. My scar was healing.

3 Months on

I could make it outside for a walk! It was excruciatingly slow and difficult. I was afraid of falling and hurting myself as well. I learned to set targets: the next lamppost, the gate, that corner, etc. Little by little, my strength, coordination, and confidence were returning. I wasn't quite running, but you have to learn to walk before you can run. My fitness instructor encouraged me and gave me the confidence to walk longer and longer distances with his support. It meant a lot to know he was there to help if I should fall.

Fatigue

As the brain heals, it needs a lot of rest. The inflammation caused by surgery or the haemorrhage disrupts the proper functioning of the brain, changing the distribution of nutrients and oxygen in and around the brain. This leads to the brain needing much more time in its repair mode, which is sleep. Often after brain surgery, a patient will sleep most of the time.

This causes muscle loss and disorientation, but as time passes and the brain heals, the patient will become less and less tired. Returning to peak energy levels is often not possible, but most people get to a level where they can live a normal life and not be exhausted all the time. It took me a few years, but I made it. Now look at me!

Six Months On

I never imagined I'd be jogging again! Hardly more than a jog, it was nevertheless an incredible freedom and sense of progress.

With this feeling of independence and hope, my thoughts turned to helping others in my situation. I knew I'd been very lucky to have the support, treatment, and guidance from my family, friends, and doctors, and I wanted to be involved in doing the same for others. I wasn't ready to go back to being a GP so I got a diploma in exercise referral and went to work for the local council, teaching others how to exercise with medical limitations—just like I'd learned. At this point, my hair was growing back and my scar was much less obvious and less painful.

Helping people in their rehabilitation after strokes or major illness was incredibly satisfying and gave me a definite sense of purpose outside my family, but I was still in a lot of pain and felt exhausted all the time. I had to learn how to limit myself. My expectations of what I could manage were still from my life before, and I had to accept I couldn't do everything I used to be able to do. This was frustrating, and I felt sad and afraid. There was always the fear of another cerebral event hanging over me. Praying to God helped and gave me direction, so too did my family. My husband kept his feelings to himself. It must have been so hard for him to see me like that.

Chronic Pain after Stroke

Many people who suffer a stroke experience chronic pain that is long-lasting or constantly recurring, and the brain damage caused by a stroke can alter the brain in a way that causes it to experience pain in different parts of the body. There is usually nothing wrong with the body but the damaged brain is misinterpreting signals, or making them up, so the sufferer often experiences excruciating pain that will not respond very well to painkillers. This is neuropathic pain that is very difficult to treat. It can feel like stabbing, burning, prickling, or numbness deep inside or on the surface of any part of the body.

As the brain heals, this pain can go away or change, but in many cases it recurs for a long time. I have chronic headaches that can be very disruptive, but they're manageable.

Two Years On

I'm running. I'm running well. The crowd of competitors has faded behind me; there are only a couple of runners ahead. Real pros, by the look of them. I want to catch them up, but I'm exhausted. I just keep pushing myself, willing myself to the finish line. The beautiful countryside passes me by as my breath and heartbeat pound in my ears. I'm going to make it. I'm running!

Out of five hundred participants in a five-mile cross-country race, I came in third. Never mind that it took me a month to fully recover. I had competed against other runners and nearly won! It was surreal and wonderful. Two years ago, I could never have seen myself even thinking about running, let alone coming in third in a race.

The chronic headaches are still the same, and I have to keep my head warm, especially in winter. It makes me grind my teeth sometimes, but I cope. My hair has grown back, and the scar is basically invisible. One of the annoying consequences of the surgery is that I can't drink alcohol anymore—not even small amounts. There are other changes as well, including subtle ones to my personality. Deep down I feel I am the person I once was, but I have to remember my limitations now and understand that I respond differently to things sometimes. I'm making progress.

Back to Work after a Stroke

Depending on the severity of the stroke, patients can be totally debilitated and unable to work or able to return to work after several days or weeks. Where the stroke appeared, how badly it occurred, and the effectiveness of treatment all affect the likelihood of someone being able to work again.

When the parts of the brain that control motor functions or eyesight are affected, it can take years of rehabilitation to rewire the brain to the point where people can do complex tasks again. In other cases where the damage is more localised or general, they can head back to work soon after.

After suffering a stroke, many people aren't allowed to drive, limiting how much they can work. I was out of work for a long time but gradually made my way back into more demanding and interesting things as I improved.

Today

My daughter is 11 now. She's beautiful and strong, and I love her so much. I am so grateful I could spend more of my life with her. I never thought I'd be part of her life again, but I'm there for her. Now I work in occupational health as a technician for as food manufacturing company. This suits my personality and gives me purpose. Being a GP again may be possible, but I feel fulfilled and happy doing what I do. I have my loving family around me and my amazing team of my GP, neuropsychologist, neuropsychiatrist, and neurologist to help me every step of the way.

My haemorrhage changed my life completely. I will never again be the person I was, but I have recovered and, more importantly, grown. It's not how I imagined my life turning out, but it has gotten better and better. Without the surgeon, I wouldn't have survived, without the doctors, I wouldn't have improved, and without my family, I wouldn't have had hope. I thank them all.

Amen.

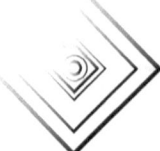

COGNITIVE CHANGES AFTER STROKE

First, when talking of cognitive changes, what does that mean? Cognition is defined as process of knowing things or thinking. In other words, as the human brain receives huge amounts of information from the surrounding environment, it has to understand, organise, and keep this information. Hence, cognition. As such, any changes in the cognition process will potentially affect how you think or know things. Bear in mind that cognition is a process which can be improved and developed. It means that some changes are positive while others are negative and even life-threatening. In this case, we are dealing with cognitive changes after a stroke. A stroke is a medical emergency that occurs when the supply of blood to the brain is reduced, cut off, or interrupted, thus depriving the brain of nutrients and oxygen. A stroke in medical terms is also referred to as a cerebrovascular accident (CVA). It is a condition defined as a dysfunction of the brain due to interruptions of the cerebral flow of blood. A stroke therefore affects the way your brain understands, stores, and organises information, thus affecting cognition.

Stroke has become the second most common cause of adult disability and death globally. However, as research in medicine and public health yields more achievements, the mortality due to stroke is decreasing. In addition, more research is now paying attention to the disabilities stroke survivors face. In most stroke cases, a myriad of cognitive changes do occur during and after stroke. Out of the approximately 15 million people suffering strokes every year, about 30 per cent end up experiencing residual disabilities. Numerous medical cases and research have shown stroke to cause cognitive impairment. However, since strokes also causes severe physical disability, they end up covering the cognitive changes; thus, post-stroke cognitive impairments can easily go unnoticed. Some of the cognitive changes which have been identified in stroke survivors include vascular dementia, aphasia, and memory loss.

A look at how a stroke affects the brain will shed light on how cognitive changes occur. As said earlier, a stroke occurs when blood supply to the brain is interfered with. The interruption of blood flow to any part can be caused by various injuries, which will be discussed later. But when the stroke occurs, the brain cells begin to die within minutes. Actually, when the brain is deprived of oxygen, it immediately begins to die and one can only retain consciousness for about two to five seconds at most. This explains why people collapse when having a stroke. Stroke-related brain damage is rather scary because the death of brain cells is irreversible. When neurons are lost or damaged, they cannot grow back. Stroke survivors thus have a high risk of experiencing permanent disability, depending on the severity of the damage, and can only recover partially. It is therefore important that stroke patients receive emergency medical attention as soon as possible to control the severity of the brain damage. This is hope. Through the right medical attention, people have survived strokes and lived to tell about them.

Types of Stroke

The cognitive changes that occur after a stroke are directly related in severity to the type of stroke and the level of the damage to the brain. A stroke can be caused by a blocked artery, a case known as ischemic stroke. A stroke can also be caused by a leaking or busted blood vessel—a haemorrhagic stroke. In other cases, the normal flow of blood to the brain may be disrupted temporarily, causing a transient ischemic attack (TIA) which may not lead to permanent brain damage, especially if the disruption lasts for a few minutes.

Depending on the type of stroke and the part of the brain deprived of nutrients and oxygen, and depending on the treatment taken, you may experience the following cognitive changes after the stroke.

Vascular Dementia

Dementia is not actually a specific disease but a term describing a combination of symptoms linked to reducing memory, among other thinking abilities. These symptoms can get severe enough to hamper a person's ability to carry out everyday activities. Vascular dementia is thus a general term describing problematic cognitive changes with planning, reasoning, memory judgement, and other thought processes due to brain damage from a stroke. Stroke does not always cause vascular dementia, but one can develop this condition when a stroke blocks an artery in the brain.

Vascular dementia is one of the most common problems after a stroke. It affects thinking abilities since the brain has a hard time processing all the information it receives. Medically speaking, post-stroke dementia (PSD) is defined by the presence of dementia three months after either a recurrent or first-time acute stroke. The risk of dementia in stroke survivors is four to twelve times higher. Vascular dementia is thus a condition occurrence due to cognitive impairments like neuronal dysfunction, neurodegenerative disorder diversity, and neuronal death. Stroke affects more than one cognitive domain, such as memory, attention, orientation, and language. The stroke impact is higher on the executive and attention functions than on memory during the time of diagnosis. Stroke can therefore cause PSD, which includes all types of dementia occurring after stroke. These include degenerative dementia like Alzheimer's disease and mixed dementia. Moreover, having vascular dementia increases the risk of a recurrent stroke.

Based on the severity, location, and size of the brain damage due to stroke, the onset of vascular dementia differs in stroke survivors. Strokes affecting the left hemisphere are more associated with vascular dementia. Some of the symptoms include confusion, memory loss, impaired motor skills, and difficulty making decisions, paying attention, planning, solving problems, or organising tasks and language problems.

Memory Loss

Loss of memory is also a cognitive change on its own. It is something that anyone can experience at any time, and this condition tends to increase with age or after a stroke. One out of three stroke survivors ends up developing memory loss. When memory loss gets sever enough to interfere with the patient's normal functioning, then it qualifies as dementia. Memory loss after stroke normally can be verbal, whereby you lose memory of stories, names, or any information that has to do with language. It can also be visual, whereby you lack or lose memory of faces, shapes, routes, or anything to be seen. Informational memory loss can also occur with the loss of memory on skills and information, making it very difficult to learn new things.

Aphasia

Aphasia is a condition very common with stroke survivors. It is characterised by having communication problems. Aphasia affects the ability to find the right words or understand what other people are saying. This difficulty also affects reading and writing. Aphasia is not a disease but a symptom of brain damage due to stroke. Different stroke survivors will experience aphasia differently. The type of aphasia will depend on the part of the brain that was damaged by the stroke. The least form of aphasia is amnesia or anomic aphasia, whereby you have difficulty using the correct names for events, things, or people. Expressive aphasia affects speech by lacking the right words to say. Receptive aphasia affects hearing, whereby one hears someone else talking or can see writings but cannot make sense of the words. The most severe type of aphasia is global aphasia, which is caused by severe and widespread damage to the language sections of the brain. Stroke survivors with global aphasia cannot express themselves through speech, reading, or writing.

Concentration Problems

During concentration, the brain screens out a lot of the other information it is receiving from around you. When a stroke affects the brain's ability to do so, concentration becomes a problem, especially in the early stages after stroke. Humans rely heavily on the brain's ability to concentrate in all thinking processes. If the brain cannot focus on something, then you cannot know how to respond to it or even remember it later.

Another cognitive change after stroke includes spatial neglect, whereby your brain, due to damages from a stroke, fails to receive information from one side of your body. When this kind of change occurs, you tend to be unaware of things in your affected side. You may not even notice that you have this problem, but it will be obvious to those around you. You may therefore find yourself missing things placed on the affected side, bumping into people, dressing only one side of your body, among other things, out of this state of inattention or neglect.

Apraxia

Apraxia is a change in cognition whereby a stroke affects your ability to plan what your body wants to do and ensure it does it the right way when you want to move. Apraxia is thus a problem of controlling or moving parts of the body. So with apraxia, moving when asked to move can be difficult, even though you do understand what you are asked to do and how to do it. Apraxia is common after stroke and is often assumed as a physical problem. With some time, however, one improves.

All the above cognitive changes tend to be worse during the first few months after the stroke. Interestingly, there are still a lot of unknowns when dealing with the brain. Essentially research has shown that the brain can form pathways between damaged neurons. Moreover, some of the sections of the brain which were not originally associated with a certain function can take over functions of the damaged parts, allowing the patient to learn afresh how to do things. For example, stroke survivors can regain motor and speech skills through therapy.

Thanks to advances in surgery, the chances of recovering from all three types of stroke are very high. In most cases, doctors may not tell exactly how well the patient will recover from the damage, but patients have oftentimes surprised doctors by exceeding the expectations.

In conclusion, not all brain damage is permanent. And these cognitive changes are likely to improve more rapidly over the first few months when the brain is most active in trying to repair itself.

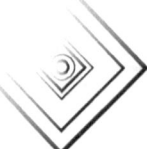

DIFFICULTIES THAT CARERS EXPERIENCE

The sudden or abrupt onset of a stroke usually results in similarly sudden life changes. Among the changes is the sudden alteration in the responsibilities and roles of the stroke survivors and their caregivers. The caregivers will have to take on multiple roles and responsibilities while the survivors temporarily or even permanently let go of important roles and responsibilities. These changes and their sudden nature have the potential to impact both the psychological and physical well-being of the stroke survivors and their caregivers.

The most stressful difficulty is the dyadic relationship problem. Due to the disruption of the interpersonal dyad between the caregiver and the patient, the caregiver may have poor communication patterns with the patient. Also, due to the reversal of roles, the caregiver may get frustrated and have intimacy issues as a result. There have been incidences whereby stroke caregivers have shown high levels of depression. Cognitive and behavioural problems, stress, patient function, family conflict, and family functioning are some of the factors associated with caregiver depression, among other negative outcomes. It is thus important to understand the nature, effectiveness, and stressfulness family stroke caregivers have to cope with during different times in the recovery trajectory.

The hospitalisation period after a stroke and the transition to home life has been identified by stroke caregivers as one of the most difficult times during the first twenty-four months of caregiving. The cognitive changes after stroke as well as the symptoms of stroke can be very stressful for caregivers. Most stroke survivors end up with long-term impairments in their psychological, cognitive, and physical functions, which are a formidable challenge to caregivers. Part of the reason why stroke caregivers exhibit elevated levels of stress is because the recipient of the care, the stroke survivor, is having a hard time processing all the information their injured brains are receiving.

As said earlier, the caregiver will have to take over roles and responsibilities they previously did not attend to. For example, if a stroke survivor suffers memory loss, the caregiver will have to take care of a patient who, although they have been taken care of and built some caregiver-recipient bond, it is torn by the cognitive changes of the stroke. The caregiver therefore has to remember everything, including things the patient used to do by herself or himself. In most cases, and sad enough, the caregiver may not understand the impact of the cognitive changes taking place in the stroke survivor. In such a case, the caregiver may consider the patient as rude, arrogant, or becoming a hard person to care for. Such scenarios may lead to the placement of the patient into nursing homes.

Mood Disturbances

This is one of the most stressful problems experienced by stroke caregivers. Mood disturbance in a stroke survivor can include anxiety and sadness. Also, many survivors exhibit depression and anxiety up to one year after the stroke, even after they have participated in the usual post-discharge programmes. When the stroke survivor shows symptoms of anxiety during non-acute and acute stages, they are usually trying to fight the fear of having a recurrent stroke. Caregivers thus have to take care of people who are moody and to some extent problematic.

For example, stroke survivors may have memory-related problems due to cognitive changes caused by damage to the brain. Such patients may therefore ask the same questions repeatedly simply because they don't remember asking earlier. They may even not recall recent events like when they last took a meal. This can be very stressful to caregivers who can even find themselves arguing with the patient.

Bowel-related problems as well as dressing difficulties are also stressful to caregivers. Essentially, stroke caregivers will find stressful to work around some of the sensory, communication, and motor problems exhibited by many stroke survivors.

In conclusion, dyadic relationship problems and interpersonal conflict are some of the difficulties caregivers experience when taking care of post-stroke patients. There is therefore a need to develop measures and interventions to manage these common yet stressful problems.

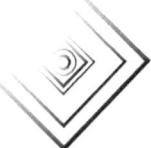

FAMILY AND FRIENDS AFTER STROKE

INTRODUCTION

According to the National Institute of Neurological Disorders and Stroke, a stroke happens when blood supply to the brain is cut or when a blood vessel in the brain suddenly bursts, spilling blood in the spaces that surround the blood cells. This can be equated to a heart attack, which is a result of a person losing blood flow to the heart whilst in the case of a stroke a person loses blood flow to the brain. This can be caused by sudden bleeding leading to what would be referred as the stroke or 'brain attack.' When blood supply to the brain is cut, the cells no longer receive oxygen and nutrients, and this is compounded by the bleeding around the cells in the brain. This results in ischemia, which means it's the loss of oxygen and nutrients to the brain (NIH 2018). Ischemia thereby leads to infarction, which refers to the death of the brain cells subsequently being replaced by cavities that are fluid filled and called infarcts.

The effects of a stroke on family and friends are considerable due to the sudden changes in personality. This is compounded by the fact that family members who may have busy schedules now become caregivers. During the first few weeks, the family will experience anxiety about the prognosis and the uncertainty that would be in the air about the future. Typically spouses of the affected victims are more likely to get into depression and emotional distress within the first few weeks of the event (Campbell, F and Gillespie, D, 2011). Other negative effects on family members include dissatisfaction with the outcomes of their lives as carers and overall anxiety. Loss of intimacy has been reported between spouses of the victims as the move from a mutually supportive relationship to one in which one takes care of the other. Challenges with the adult children are common as they struggle to cope with taking care of their children and their parents. The psychological distress and decreased quality of life in caring for the patient is more prominent in women as opposed to men (Campbell, F and Gillespie, D, 2011). Stroke has the effect of altering how families lead their lives as carers are unable to do half of their usual activities after a stroke survivor has returned from hospital. The family relationship after a stroke tends to deteriorate with significant family dysfunction within nine months after a stroke. A study (by Clark et al. 2004) showed that 32 per cent of the families affected by a stroke were reported to be dysfunctional with 66 per cent experience conflict within their ranks. Stroke has the effect of the patient losing friends (according to Northcott, S and Hilari, K, 2011). The loss in friends is usually due to reduced energy, physical disability, changing social desires, and the ultimate loss of activities the patient and the friends shared.

Families Giving up Work to Look after a Spouse

The devastating effect of some strokes means that the patient needs to be taken care of as they are in a disabled state. Some spouses may have to give up work in order to take care of the patient. This puts a strain on the spouse, especially if they are women, mostly due to the dissatisfaction brought about by their lives being reduced to those of a caregiver (Campbell, F and Gillespie, D, 2011). Even though it's usually a tough decision, some spouses opt for this especially when they are older as they are usually near retirement and because the children are all grown up. The decision is better for most overcare facilities. The types of rehabilitation options available for recovering stroke patients vary from inpatient rehabilitation facilities to outpatient rehabilitation programmes.

Most stroke patients remain in hospital in the early days of the stroke for two to three weeks to participate in intensive rehabilitation programmes. Whilst decisions are being made at home of the need for therapy and twenty-four-hour access to nursing support. The home and outpatient programmes offer patients the option to travel to hospital for specialised care or to receive the care from home, where a specialist will visit the home to provide therapy. Governments have not taken special concerns to stroke rehabilitation and family support as they have with cancer and other illnesses.

Home Changes after Stroke

The home environment can play a crucial role to the recovery of the patient. Some modifications need to be done so as to accommodate the patient's limitations as the patient may be in a wheelchair. The home environment that may need to be changed will include the social and cultural environment as well as the physical aspects of the home, such as the layout (Stroke Center 2019). It's imperative that the home be adapted to suit the recovery of the stroke victim. This would involve changes to the stairs where a ramp would be installed to enable the patient to use the wheelchair. The bathroom can be installed with grab bars to help provide the victim with somewhere to hold as the patients often have difficulty walking and standing (Stroke Center 2019). Additionally, smart devices which can detect when the victims fall in the bathrooms can be installed to enhance their safety. Shower doors can also be replaced with shower curtains. In the toilet, technology-assisted toilets can be deployed to wash and dry the perineal region, thereby improving the independence for patients (Jeffrey, J et al. 2017). Lighting should be adjusted such that all the switches for all rooms can be fitted at one place for easy access by the stroke patient. For bathtubs, they can be modified by installing a transfer tub bench, which is a seating device that extends beyond the side of the tap to enable the stroke patient to slide into the tab rather than step in. The furniture in the home can be repositioned to give more space for the patient to move around. If the patient can use the stairs, though not recommended, side rails should be installed if they aren't already there. The patient can also have a nurse call system installed in his or her bedroom.

Conclusion

Strokes are a very serious condition and can take a toll on the patient, family, and friends, leading to significant changes in lives of both the caregivers and the patient. The strain is significant on finances as there is home altering coupled with underfunded rehabilitation centres and the need to have family take care of the stroke survivor. With all this, it is important to be well prepared when it comes to taking care of a loved one by having comprehensive knowledge and avoiding situations that may put you or the stroke survivor at further risk.

I received a lot of prayers from friends and family all round the world. The words were comforting.

The extent of the brain damage became clear a few years later following my arrest. My family felt it was a great toll on my husband and provided support for my family as best they could.

I will always be grateful for the ongoing support I receive.

As time progresses, the true impact of my cerebral events come alight as I struggle with behavioural problems. Some distant family member concluded that I had been exposed to Satan and must have done something very bad for this to be my punishment.

I recognised the cultural issues that my rare disease presented and the perceptions of some relatives. The incidence of infectious diseases in my home country is high, and I suppose that crossed the minds of some people. I was young and had a stroke. These symptoms are associated with other infectious diseases so the empathy for younger victims with illness/death is limited.

It was five years later that the real extent of my illness became evident to my close family. As I battled to be a wife, daughter, doctor, and mother, I couldn't multitask anymore. I was broken, and no one understood. My husband concentrated on maintaining my daughter's routine. I was no one anymore. My career gave me the self-confidence to feel like a worthwhile member of society. After this was taken away from me, my battle to regain my medical licence left me depressed and withdrawn.

I knew the prognosis of my illness, and only if it was explained did others have their own picture.

That is the problem with mental health in developing countries. It is rarely recognised.

Finally after nineteen years of marriage, after behavioural changes that my immediate family could no longer cope, with we decided to separate.

References

NIH. (2018). *Stroke: Hope Through Research,* https://www.ninds.nih.gov/Disorders/Patient-Caregiver-Education/Hope-Through- Research/Stroke-Hope-Through-Research#1105_1

Campbell, F and Gillespie, D. (2011). Effect of stroke on family carers and family relationships https://www.researchgate.net/publication/51704653_Effect_of_stroke_on_family_carers_and_family_relationships

Clark et al. (2004). *Influence of stroke survivor characteristics and family conflict surrounding recovery on caregivers' mental and physical health.* https://www.ncbi.nlm.nih.gov/pubmed/15586137

Northcott, S and Hilari, K. (2011). *Why do people lose their friends after a stroke?* https://www.ncbi.nlm.nih.gov/pubmed/21899670

Horn. (2009). *Hospital-based stroke rehabilitation in the United States.*, https://www.ncbi.nlm.nih.gov/pubmed/19443346

American Stroke Association. (2019). *Choosing the Right Stroke Rehab Facility,* https://www.strokeassociation.org/en/life-after-stroke/stroke-rehab/choosing-the-right- stroke-rehab-facility

Stroke center. (2019). *Adapting the Home after a Stroke* http://www.strokecenter.org/patients/caregiver-and-patient-resources/home-modification/adapting-the-home-after-a-stroke/

Jeffrey, J et al. (2017). *Technology-assisted toilets: Improving independence and hygiene in stroke rehabilitation,* https://journals.sagepub.com/doi/full/10.1177/2055668317725686

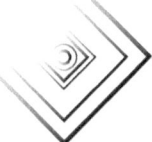

Cultural Differences in Psychiatry

Psychiatric illnesses and other mental disorders as well as their psychosocial disabilities form a significant source of morbidity and a huge drain to national resources. According to the World Health Organization, some of the most common mental disorders prevail in both the developing and developed world. Most of the 400 million people suffering from psychiatric morbidity come from developing countries, where only a few of them can access mental healthcare. In the same developing countries, especially a greater part of Africa, there are certain beliefs associated with the cause and treatment of mental illnesses, which is part of the reason why some people do not practise formal mental health services.

Psychiatric illnesses attack without discrimination. They do not distinguish among socioeconomic status, level of education, race, culture, or gender, yet the type of treatment and opinion you receive as a mental illness patient will always have a cultural bias. A perfect example is in the traditional African society in which there are strong and prevalent beliefs in not only the existence but also the involvement of ancestral spirits, diviners, sorcerers, and witches who can influence a person's well-being by subtly manipulating certain agents that make up a person's psychosocial environment. As a result of these beliefs, such societies have a high tendency to attribute life's misfortunes, such as ill health, particularly psychiatric illness, and death to activities by said supernatural agents. Studies dating as far back as the 1950s show that cultures inclined to such beliefs classify the ultimate pathway or cause of mental illness and disequilibrium from supernatural afflictions into either simple bewitchment or malignant bewitchment. A simple bewitchment is where the subject came into direct contact with a charm or amulet which had been doctored by either a witch or sorcerer. For a malignant bewitchment, the subject develops the obsessive and strong belief that he or she is bewitched (Field 1955). Many recent studies show that the implementation of alternative practices of treating mental illnesses in African countries do have an important role to play. In the same way that some African cultures and societies believe that mental illness is caused by supernatural powers like witchcraft and sorcery, they believe in the use of the same agents for the treatment of psychiatric illnesses. As such, traditional experts like healers, witches, and religious advisors are sought to provide alternative healthcare that is different from Western medicine. Furthermore, these witches and traditional healers tend to be more affordable and accessible compared to the Western type of healthcare. Witchcraft is a traditional spiritual concept together with other supernatural phenomena like sorcery, spirit possession, and bewitchment (Dhadphale 2015).

Culturally appropriate treatment of psychiatric illnesses comes in many shapes and sizes, but all imply a supernatural context. For instance, diviners and traditional healers specialise in the use of divination to perform some kind of diagnosis on the subject. They can divine the cause of the mental illness. In one case from Uganda which was featured in the BBC in 2015, Joseph Atukunda narrates how witchcraft and traditional healers saved his life. Joseph was suicidal after losing a battle with deep depression, but right before he took rat poison or hanged himself, he had something like a vision telling him he could find help. As he narrates, he is very clear he does not know from whom the vision came, whether it was Krishna, Jesus, Muhammad, or Buddha. However, according to Western medical terms, Joseph was suffering from a severe case of mental illness called bipolar affective disorder which gave him severe mood swings, taking him from despair to elation. His condition would last for weeks or even months. Despite the challenge of getting psychiatric attention in Uganda, which has about thirty psychiatrists against 35 million people, Joseph was lucky enough to be admitted at Butabika, which was the only psychiatric healthcare centre in the country. The WHO estimated that 90 per cent of people suffering from mental illness never get treatment (BBC 2015).

A psychiatric hospital can be a tough place, especially in Africa where they are stigmatised. People with mental illnesses actually prefer to hide their condition, because if admitted to a psychiatric hospital, they are perceived to have been bewitched or to have done something evil enough to have angered the ancestors who in return struck them with the psychiatric illness. The hospital helped Joseph get through some of his toughest and most manic episodes when he became violent and was even put in isolation. Sometimes he would be stripped naked to be given the medication. Joseph admits that even though the hospital has made improvements with regards to Western healthcare services, psychiatric hospitals should rely much less on medication. The fact that he had to take medication every single day was a constant reminder that he was sick—a mind-set nobody would want.

Part of the greater challenge with psychiatric illnesses is that they can easily be misunderstood. The human brain remains an unsolvable puzzle, and in a similar way, most disorders are a mystery. Western medication has come a long way to address either the signs or symptoms associated with mental illnesses, and medicines even try to make the life of the patient significantly closer to their normal life before they got sick. In Uganda, psychiatrists estimate that more than 90 per cent of the population believes psychiatric illnesses are directly linked to demons or curses, which are witchcraft. Joseph agrees with this deduction. He indeed spent time with a traditional healer who, using divine and mysterious means, diagnosed him by telling him that witchcraft was involved in his misfortune. He had demons in his head, and the doctor had to make a cut on Joseph's head to put in the traditional medicine. In addition, the traditional healer slaughtered a cock and washed him in the blood.

Although the methods used by the traditional healer were crude, it saved his life and thus witchcraft had a bigger role to play in his mental healthcare. Joseph was treated and is now well after the spiritual healer's crude intervention. Joseph is one among many African people who cannot discard witchcraft and spiritual healers as people who cannot contribute at all to mental wellness (BBC 2015).

Generally, any idea of the supernatural is omnipresent, but very few Western psychiatrists can write a report of spiritual and demon possession. The link between psychiatric illnesses and various forms of witchcraft is undeniable. In Zambia, for example, a woman called Maria was locally known as a witch who practised witchcraft and was believed to accomplish supernatural things like making people disappear. While that may not be proved, she was arrested and charged for kidnapping a young girl by using witchcraft. One of the people in her defence was Manohar Dhadphale, a psychiatrist who had knowledge about the spiritual framework of Zambia. The 56-year-old Maria came from a society that believed witchcraft exists and affects people mentally and physically; it is not an imagination. This same society agreed that Western medical practices did not really understand witchcraft and therefore ought to refer victims to traditional healers and witches who are able to lift the curse or bewitchment and treat spirit possession.

After closer observation upon admission to a psychiatric centre, Maria turned out to have been suffering from a chronic case of schizophrenia and was in a defective state. Her witchcraft was due to a past relapse during which she would boast of her supernatural prowess. The Zambian court was more inclined to believe that Maria should be charged for using witchcraft to kidnap a girl than it was to believe that she was mentally ill. This case goes a long way to show that, indeed, there exists a relationship between mental illness and witchcraft, but with a difference in the Western and African perspective of each. Researchers like Prince (1964) suggest that traditional healers should play a role in dealing with spirit passion cases. In Kenya for example, it was found that a significant number of mental illness patients seeking psychiatric services had also sought traditional healers (Dhadphale 2015). It therefore seems that psychiatric illnesses have two angles: the conventional Western approach and the spiritual and traditional witchcraft approach. One should explore either depending on one's belief and spiritual or religious stand and conviction.

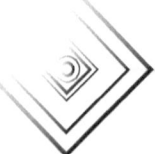

RACISM IN PSYCHIATRY

The cultural factors on psychiatry illnesses run so deep. *The Guardian* has reported that black people among the minority ethnic people are usually shortchanged when it comes to mental health services *(The Guardian* 2015). Among the reported cases is one of Ramone, a black immigrant in the UK. When he developed a severe mental illness, he required long-term care, but his case was not eligible for treatment. This meant that when he became extremely ill, he was sectioned, mostly by the police, and would be admitted to the mental health unit and medicated till he could be released. This was the procedure for more than five years.

People from black communities or other minority ethnic backgrounds are very likely to be subjected to some crisis mental healthcare. This inequality is usually due to racism, stigma, and poor mental health services. Crisis care like sectioning makes the patients find the care not to be working for them. Ramone's experience is one among dozens that have been collected by the Race Equality Foundation. Sectioning, especially due to racism, leaves the patients disempowered. They cannot even feel that the people and staff who sectioned them would be caring or compassionate enough.

References

Field MJ. (1955) Witchcraft as a primitive interpretation of mental disorder. *J Ment Sci*1955;**101**: 826–33. Retrieved on June 13, 2019 from: https://mh.bmj.com/content/30/1/23#ref-5

Dhadphale M. (2015). A witch defended by a psychiatrist. *BJPsych international*, *12*(2), 49–50. Retrieved on June 13, 2019 from: https://www.ncbi.nlm.nih.gov/pmc/articles/PMC5618918/

The Guardian (2015). Black and Minority Ethnic People are Shortchanged by Mental Health Services. Retrieved on June 13, 2019 from: https://www.theguardian.com/healthcare-network/2015/jun/25/black-minority-ethnic-people-shortchanged-mental-health-services

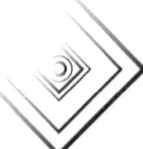

CRIMINAL CONVICTIONS AND BRAIN INJURY

> There are risks associated with her impulsive behavior in a range of situations, including driving, putting herself in a vulnerable positions, aggression towards others, particularly after a relatively small amounts of alcohol ...
> —*Neuropsychiatrist*

Is there a link between criminal convictions and brain injuries? This is one of the highly researched questions in both the legal and medical fields. Numerous studies have been conducted elucidating a connection between what is termed as traumatic brain injury and criminal behaviour and criminal convictions. Previous studies have shown beyond reasonable doubt that there are several factors to criminal behaviour and traumatic brain injury (TBI)/acquired brain injury (ABI).

Brain injury is a great cause of disability and even death among children. TBI/ABI generally compromises important brain functions that deal with social behaviour and self-regulation to the extent that it makes you more susceptible to behavioural disorders and even psychiatric morbidity. Crime, especially in young people, has become a great social issue. And most of the people who begin as early starters of criminal behaviour end up continuing in that same behaviour—and even worse—for a lifetime. Despite the numerous other factors playing a role, brain injury is a risk factor which is characteristic in earlier and violent criminal offences. It is therefore important to understand whether indeed brain injury increases the likelihood that a person will commit a crime. Potential injury factors should be considered when dealing with people who are accused of crime (Schofield et al. 2015).

Crime presents substantial costs. While most criminal behaviour peaks during early adulthood and late adolescence, most prolific offenders like the early starters end up committing up to 77 per cent of crimes. Considering a single prolific criminal, his or her lifetime costs of crime can range from 1 to 2 million euros. The criminal correction system, on the other hand, may seem to be failing, especially when 73 per cent of people below 18 years and 47 per cent of adults end up being reconvicted within the first years of release. In England, for example, criminal offences by ex-prisoners cost approximately 10 to 13 billion euros every year. This explains why in recent times the call to improve both the physical and mental health of prisoners has intensified, in the hope that it will reduce crime.

Leading theories in the crime and brain injury relationships suggest that antisocial behaviour, difficult temperaments, and neuropsychological deficits lead to certain problems in life which are linked to crime. Brain injuries, which tend to be very common among young people, have been shown to cause personality and cognitive issues, which possibly increase a person's risks of engaging in criminal behaviour. The other view is that traumatic brain/acquired brain injuries are very common among young people and often cause personality and cognitive issues which increase the risk of engaging in crime. This apparent link between brain injuries and crime is quite complex.

Research by Turkstra, Jones, and Toler in 2003 tested the hypothesis that traumatic brain injury is associated with violent crime. Their work admits that there are several research studies suggesting the TBI and crime linkage and even cited a report where 50 per cent of people with traumatic brain injury were convicted of crimes while only 5 to 15 per cent were convicted without TBI. Another report found that out of sixteen death row inmates, twelve of them had a history of brain damage, mostly due to injuries from insults inflicted by caregivers. There was also a study carried out on 279 Vietnam veterans with TBI who showed higher ratings of aggression, violence, hostility, and anger compared to those *without* brain injury.

Despite these numerous and many more examples of a link between brain injury and violence, Turkstra et al. (2003) argue that the supposed link between crime and brain injury is just an epiphenomenon and that the incidences of both criminal behaviour and brain injury are influenced by underlying demographic variables. Therefore, criminal behaviour, especially violent crime, according to Turkstra et al., is more likely due to a complex interaction of various factors like genetic predisposition, poverty, stress, child abuse, and substance abuse. At a young age, people who are raised in abusive and impoverished environments end up missing on such pro-social behaviours and thus are more likely to commit crime and engage in activities that put their brains at risk of injuries.

The alternative view which is supported by more research is that traumatic and acquired brain injuries damage the frontal lobe. The frontal lobe, which is associated with controlling the limbic and subcortical structures involved in making *primitive impulses,* gets compromised. *Lesions in the frontal lobe area influence various functions like self-control, social perception, making judgement, moods, and emotions.*

The link between brain injury and criminal activity reflects brain-injury-related cognitive and emotional impairments on a person's behaviour. This even explains why people with traumatic/acquired brain injury may *wrongly perceive situations.* For examples, they may interpret sarcasm as a threat, make poor social judgements, conduct themselves inappropriately in public, and lack communications skills to assist in negotiating conflicts verbally. They may also overreact to stimuli. Such behaviour has been observed in both adults and children with brain injuries, especially to the frontal lobe lesions. Hence, the link that brain injury leads to criminal behaviour (Williams et al. 2018).

Brain injury in this context refers to an insult to the brain due to an external mechanical force like a blow to the head from an assault, a car crash, or a fall. Essentially, these are injuries that can cause lacerations and bruising to various structures of the brain, particularly around the bony protrusions on the basal surface of the skull. Internal bleedings and secondary hypoxia resulting from injuries can damage the brain further, by breaking the flow of oxygen and nutrients to some parts of the brain. The severity of a brain injury can be determined by the Glasgow Coma Scale. Out of a maximum of 15, 13 denotes mild, 9–12 is moderate, and severe is for a score of 8 and below. The loss of consciousness (LOC) or post-traumatic amnesia can also gauge the severity of a brain injury.

A mild traumatic brain injury involves an LOC of zero to thirty minutes. It is moderate to severe when it's thirty minutes and over. The mildest injuries are considered concussions which cause some disorientation of time and a brief or no loss of consciousness. Such injuries rarely cause permanent changes to the brain. The risk of chronic problems increases with increased severity. With moderate and severe brain injuries, you are more likely to have long-term behavioural, neurocognitive, and psychiatric disturbances (Williams et al. 2018)

One case which sheds more light on the link between brain injury and crime is that of Aaron Hernandez back in 2017. This former tight end football player for the New England Patriots was convicted for murdering another football player who was dating his fiancée's sister. He was also charged with shooting and killing two other men in 2017. Aaron later committed suicide in his prison cell. This is a perfect case of violent criminal behaviour, and with the death of the perpetrator, a closure had to be reached. A team of researchers from Boston University was tasked with examining Aaron's brain.

As it turned out, the researchers reported that Aaron suffered from the most severe case of chronic traumatic encephalopathy for a person his age. What Aaron had was a progressive degenerative disease of the brain that is mostly common in individuals with a history of multiple brain trauma. Of course, legal experts using their customary scientific caution tried not to connect Aaron's brain pathology to his crime. But stating the facts as they are, Aaron's severe brain injuries would have led him to making poor judgements and impulse controls which are hallmarks of the criminal behaviour that landed him in life imprisonment. If his brain got this badly damaged during his years playing football, then his condition is a partial explanation for his criminal actions. The same needs to be extended to the millions of prisoners suffering from an extensive and unrecognised health problem of brain injury (Bozelko 2017).

Brain injury, especially among children and young people, is a real and huge cause of morbidity and mortality. It has been referred to as the silent epidemic since social and healthcare professionals do not recognise it. Williams et al. (2018) provide a thorough research into the link between brain injuries and crime. Their findings show that TBI is associated with a high risk of committing crime. Birth cohorts, those who had brain injuries at young ages or adolescence, were four times more likely to have a mental disorder coupled with a coexisting offence in adulthood. Studies on data linkage and populations are also consistent, indicating that brain injuries increase criminality (Schofield et al. 2015). Traumatic brain/acquired injury at the very least should serve as a marker for various issues that indicate the risk of crime, even though evidence from a broad range of populations and age groups indicates that TBI is independently a risk factor of crime.

In conclusion, there has been a previous assumption that traumatic/acquired brain injury is just another coincidental phenomenon or occurrence in risk takers or people whose premorbid live trajectory was set towards crime. But much recent research suggests otherwise. Addressing brain injuries will not only improve the lives of the offenders but will also crucially reduce crime.

My Forensic History

On 10 September 2016, I drank a small amount of alcohol and took codeine to relieve my constant pain. Then I went to a local pub to meet a friend.

I cannot remember much about the rest of the events, but I found myself in custody for twenty-four hours facing charges of common assault.

My brain injury, painkillers, and alcohol were major mitigation factors on the verdict. I received a fine of £300 from the magistrates' court.

I remain very remorseful for an action I can barely remember and for any harm I had caused.

Custody is not the environment I am familiar with, and suffering from claustrophobia made it worse. The night in custody followed by an emergency admission to the hospital made me reflect on improving my mental condition. I was referred for neurorehabilitation, which helped me address my problems.

Following the severe offence, I had to undergo further evaluation of the state of my brain, particularly the frontal lobe.

MR angiogram suggested further ischaemic changes from my previous scans in 2012, the status of my anterior circulation vasculopathy related.

I was referred back to my neurosurgeon for consideration of a bypass—this time on the right side. Further investigations confirmed the MRI findings, but I did not require further surgery at this stage.

References

Bozelko (2017). Traumatic brain injury should be a factor when judging individuals accused of crimes. Retrieved on 18

June 19, 2019 from https://www.statnews.com/2017/12/07/traumatic-brain-injury-crime/

Schofield, P. W., Malacova, E., Preen, D. B., D'Este, C., Tate, R., Reekie, J., ... Butler, T. (2015). Does Traumatic Brain Injury Lead to Criminality? A Whole-Population Retrospective Cohort Study Using Linked Data. *PloS one*, *10*(7), e0132558. doi:10.1371/journal.pone.0132558. Retrieved on 18 June 19, 2019 from https://www.ncbi.nlm.nih.gov/pmc/articles/PMC4501545/

Turkstra, Lyn & Jones, D & L Toler, Hon. (2003). Brain injury and violent crime. Brain injury : [BI]. 17. 39-47. 10.1080/0269905021000010122. Retrieved on 18 June 19, 2019 from https://www.researchgate.net/publication/10957425_Brain_injury_and_violent_crime

Williams, W. H., Chitsabesan, P., Fazel, S., McMillan, T., Hughes, N., Parsonage, M., & Tonks, J. (2018). Traumatic brain injury: a potential cause of violent crime?. *The lancet. Psychiatry*, *5*(10), 836–844. doi:10.1016/S2215-0366(18)30062-2. Retrieved on 18 June 19, 2019 from https://www.ncbi.nlm.nih.gov/pmc/articles/PMC6171742/

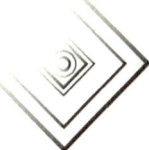

FATIGUE AFTER STROKE (POST-STROKE FATIGUE)

Everyone gets tired after having a busy day, working for long hours on a certain task, or even lacking sleep. But unlike the normal tiredness one experiences, the level and kind of fatigue for a stroke survivor is different. Stroke survivors experience what can be termed as overwhelming fatigue, both mentally and physically. This kind of fatigue also happens to be one of the most common symptoms after a stroke. Interestingly, this type of fatigue is not in any way related to the quality of sleep one receives or the level of activity one engages in (NSA 2019). This type of stroke may not improve with rest. It is, however, important to really understand and manage this kind of fatigue, especially as a stroke survivor or as someone looking after a stroke survivor (Stroke Association 2019)

Getting tired is actually a very normal aspect of life and the human brain, and it happens for all sorts of reasons like lack of sleep. Usually just resting, relaxing, and getting some sleep helps alleviate such tiredness. Post-stroke fatigue is, however, different. Apart from the fact that it is not like typical fatigue, post-stroke fatigue comes with a great feeling of lack of strength and energy, to the point where one feels extremely weary and tired even when one has not engaged in any recent energy-demanding activity. Post-stroke fatigue usually comes a short time after a mild or severe stroke. Most definitions of this kind of fatigue from stroke survivors have one thing in common. The fatigue entails a period of at least two weeks or a period shortly after the stroke where one experiences a lack of energy as well as an increased need to rest nearly every day. This fatigue usually makes it hard for one to engage in day-to-day activities (Stroke Association 2019).

One might be tempted to ignore and dismiss this feeling of fatigue after stroke. One may decide to stoically carry on with one's activities despite the fatigue. However, by ignoring post-stroke fatigue, a stroke survivor can be storing up future problems by not giving themselves the best chance to recover. One ought to remember that the occurrence of a stroke greatly interferes with the normal functioning and health of the brain and the brain needs every opportunity it can get to recover and repair the damage (Stroke Association 2019).

Post-stroke survivors should, however, not be worried because post-stroke fatigue is not an isolated matter. More than half of all post-stroke survivors experience post-stroke fatigue. The only problem is that post-stroke fatigue presents as an invisible symptom and many people are likely to ignore it.

Actually most people confuse post-stroke with feeling tired, but unlike typical tiredness, post-stroke fatigue comes without warning. This stroke makes someone feel unwell and like one is losing control of one's recovery. Post-stroke fatigue is very common among stroke survivors. Various research studies on fatigue after stroke reveal that some stroke survivors find themselves always feeling tired and more people are sometimes tired. Another research done twelve months after stroke reported that 50 per cent of stroke survivors cited tiredness as their main problem. One is therefore more likely to experience post-stroke fatigue shortly after stroke when the brain is initiating the recovery process (Stroke Association 2019).

Post-fatigue is not related to the type or severity of the stroke. This means that post-stroke fatigue usually ranges from mild to severe, but the intensity of the stroke fatigue due to haemorrhagic stroke is just as common as those caused by ischaemic strokes. But one is more likely to experience fatigue after a stroke than after a mini stroke/TIA. Post-stroke fatigue can remain a problem, even after making a full recovery.

According to some research studies, older people and women who suffered from fatigue before the stroke are more likely to experience post-stroke fatigue. Other studies show that younger individuals who were previously totally fit can also experience fatigue after stroke. There are also some individual studies which draw a connection between being unemployed and experiencing post-stroke fatigue. Such a relationship is not yet clear and needs more research.

For most stroke survivors, fatigue is the most upsetting and difficult issue they have to cope with after stroke. Fatigue prevents someone from engaging fully in rehabilitation because one always feels so tired and non-energetic. One may eventually be unable to regain one's independence in everyday activities, thus making it difficult to go back to work, socialise again, or even enjoy day-to-day activities. Moreover, post-stroke fatigue can greatly affect quality of relationships and life, especially since friends and family may not be familiar with post-stroke.

Post-stroke fatigue usually leads to the question of why someone feels so tired. This fatigue is likely brought about by a mixture of emotional and physical factors. The exact reason why people who have experienced stroke have fatigue while others don't is not fully known. The main reason given for post-stroke fatigue is massive cerebral insult and needing to recover. Another likely scenario is that, in the weeks and months after stroke, the process of the body healing and being rehabilitated can take up a lot of energy.

There are also other factors that affect how tired one feels after stroke. For example if one has sleeping problems like insomnia or some sleep-related breathing disorder, eating problems, or an underactive thyroid gland after stroke, then one may experience a higher level of tiredness. Some medications can bring about fatigue. One good example is beta blocker drugs taken for high blood pressure and heart problems. Medications for epilepsy, antidepressants, and pain relievers can all cause fatigue. Some researchers have also suggested that fatigue is related to inflammatory cells and hormones which are usually disturbed by stroke (NSA 2019).

Treatment

There is no particular medication for the treatment of post-stroke fatigue, but there are a lot of procedures to manage this condition. First, *get a proper diagnosis* to find out if there is any other co-morbidity causing fatigue, such as underactive thyroid or anaemia. A general practitioner or a specialist stroke nurse can also check if there are pertinent medical conditions or medications that can be causing the fatigue. Doctors should keep reviewing the medications of stroke survivors to see if the fatigue is a side effect of the medication, such as amitriptyline and beta blockers. Try not to stop taking a medication suddenly without consultation with your doctor, even if you suspect it is making you feel tired (NSA 2019).

Managing fatigue is recommended, especially if one intends to go back to work after stroke. Fatigue is actually referred to as one of the invisible disabilities. Managing fatigue helps with emotional problems like frustration and practical problems like inactivity and reduced social life (NSA 2019).

Post-stroke survivors ought to remember that fatigue is very common and it is not their fault. As an invisible impairment, fatigue may not be obvious to other people, and they may not understand how you feel. If you get back to work, fatigue may be interpreted as laziness or loss of interest in work. In an effort to return to work, consideration should be made for a phased return. You can get help from occupational therapists and your doctor. Try not to push yourself too much, and keep a record of how you feel each day to monitor your progress. Post-stroke can be very upsetting, but knowing it is due to the stroke is a step in the right direction (NSA 2019).

My Experience with Post-Stroke Fatigue

The first three weeks after my brain haemorrhage were awful. I had a headache affecting the back of my head and radiating to my neck. I couldn't move my head freely. It was terrible.

Associated with nausea, I thought I was going to die soon. I was given Oramorph for severe pain, but that left me tired, scared, and anxious.

After four weeks, I was able to talk better, and my cognition was improving. My mood was still very low and scared.

I was transferred to a specialist hospital to see a neurosurgeon and discuss my poor perfusion to my frontal lobe. My neurosurgeon arranged for me to have pre- and post-Acetazolamide SPECT scans together with a further MRI scanning and BOLD reactivity. This confirmed bilateral reduction in cerebral vascular. Despite being a doctor, I did not like the sound of any of it. I was in denial?

I went on to have a left, medium-flow, STA-2 bypass. Yes, that's what the doctor said. My superficial temporal artery was in good calibre to be a donor. As I faced ten-hour pioneering vascular surgery that I had never heard of, my hands were in the hands on my doctors. I had no control over this. I was terrified! So now the front of my brain is supplied by the artery from the side of my face. This was my invisible experience as a doctor and a patient.

After brain surgery, it took me at least two years to feel half normal. I enjoyed running pre-stroke, and that was my postoperative aim. I think my cardiovascular fitness has improved my cerebral circulation as well as the donor temporal artery, which matures with time—like a nice block of cheese.

I was tired all the time. I still cannot multitask. I leave chores unfinished, but I don't remember starting them.

References

Stroke Association (2019). Fatigue after Stroke. Retrieved on 26 June 2019 from https://www.stroke.org.uk/sites/default/files/fatigue_after_stroke.pdf

National Stroke Association NSA (2019). Fatigue. Retrieved on 26 June 2019 from https://www.stroke.org/we-can-help/survivors/stroke-recovery/post-stroke-conditions/physical/fatigue/

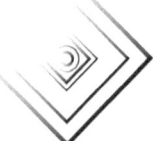

Going Back to Work after Stroke

In the unfortunate event that someone suffers a stroke while in the prime of life, during the recovery the thought of whether you can return to work can be challenging. After a stroke, blood flow to the brain is cut off and as a result some brain cells die, causing potential health effects like balance issues, paralysis (difficulty in movement), and communicating problems (dysphasia). This includes how you speak, your ability to understand what is being said, and your reading and writing skills. However, despite the myriad of challenges that a stroke survivor may encounter, going back to work is actually a good way to enhance the recovery process. Stroke survivors can actually go back to work with the right care, advice, and support.

Various research has suggested that working is healthy and not working is one of the risk factors of stroke (Westerlind et al. 2017). Work brings a certain form of satisfaction, especially when one's life before the stroke revolved around work. For example, most people have built their social life around their work. Work is what occupies most of their twenty-four hours in a day, whether it's taking care of their family, attending to patients, or even operating a machinery in a factory. Work is an essential part of what makes up people's lives. As a result, the impacts of stroke affect every aspect of a person's life and work. Stroke survivors who are not able to return to work are likely to get *depressed*, be less satisfied with life, and live in isolation with a reduced quality of life.

Stroke has for long been associated with people who are retired from work. But 20 per cent of strokes occur in younger people. When most people think about stroke survivors, they think of someone who is paralyzed and bedridden with difficulty walking. While there are some severe strokes, the disability strokes, employers should realise that when someone suffers a stroke, it does not mean that they are incapacitated or cannot go back to doing the job they did before. Stroke is more of an individualised phenomenon. Going back to work will depend on the seriousness of the stroke and nature of the effects.

Stroke brings about impairments, and different people take different amounts of time to recover. A person with a broken hand may be back to full working condition after six weeks, but a stroke survivor needs an extended time to recover before they can return to work. Usually most employers are not aware that recovering from stroke can take eight months or longer. People who suffer from a mild stroke may not necessarily exhibit severe impacts like speech and paralysis problems and thus are more likely to recovery sooner and get back to work. People's ability to return to work after a stroke, as well as how long it will take them depends greatly on the effects of the stroke, what work they were doing before the stroke, and the kind of support their employer is willing to give them. Of course going back to work does not have to be at the previous position one was in, with the same roles and responsibilities. Stroke survivors can still be back to work even if they are not doing the exact same job they did before. There are various options through which a stroke survivor can remain productive.

It is the legal responsibility of the employer to ensure that the stroke does not stop stroke survivors from keeping their job. In this regard, the employer should do all they can to ensure that stroke survivors receives the same access and rights to opportunities as they did before the stroke. Stroke survivors, especially those who had been working in a certain job position, should probably retain their specialty or position. Employers can also benefit from stroke survivors who come back to work. Such employees usually know the job in its entirety, know the environment, the routine, and the staff, and thus are likely to be more successful in their previous job than in a new one. As such, employers should do all they can to ensure that a person does not lose their job and that their position is not filled after a stroke.

Working in a familiar environment is a recommended step to enable the stroke survivor to regain their brain functionality before the stroke. It becomes easier for the survivor to relearn tasks and memorise routines the brain was used to. The same applies to post-stroke employees who may have problems with eye-body coordination.

According to the 2018 American Stroke Association's International Stroke Conference held in Los Angeles, researchers analysed the study of 252 stroke survivors who were in their working age. The researchers found that stroke patients who had jobs before and after suffering their first stroke were more likely to have healthier minds two years after the stroke, compared to those who didn't go back to work. Returning to work after stroke is thus associated with a lower risk of cognitive decline. Going back to work is essential to recovering from stroke and is vital to some individuals. Going back to work, psychologically speaking, hinges on the stimulation of the brain to help it create and replace damaged neural pathways necessary for the improvement of neurological functions (Castaneda 2018).

Post-stroke employees need to work out their return-to-work formula with their employer and occupational therapist. By doing so, employers and occupational therapists can suggest tools which will enable the stroke survivor to overcome stroke-related speech and motor limitations. Such tools include sit-stand workstations, speech recognition software, computer keyboards usable with one hand, and special gloves that strengthen the grip. In as much as it is good to return to work after a stroke, it should not be done in a manner that compromises on safety.

Most employees and employers are unaware of certain invisible impairments. A 2016 study from the Queen Mary University of London and the University of Cambridge found that most stroke survivors who return to work were greatly challenged by invisible impairments like fatigue and concentration problems. In the study, sixty post-stroke workers reported that apart from their physical impairments, they suffered more from impairments which are not physically noticeable. Impairments like memory issues and change in personality potentially threatened their job. Invisible impairments in stroke survivors who return to work can be easily misunderstood by the employer, stroke survivor, and even the general practitioner since they are not obvious. The study suggests that a successful return-to-work formula for a stroke survivor should entail adjustments like shorter working hours, a possibility of working from home, and a gradual return to the work environment. Stroke survivors may try to work beyond their capability to fight the fear and worry that they may not be able to get back to their previous working condition. As such, their employers, doctors, and occupational therapists should have great knowledge on the potential issues that the patient could encounter when they return to work.

The decision to return to work should not be left to the stroke survivor alone. The employer, doctors, worker, and occupational therapist should help determine whether a survivor is in a position to return to work. A mention earlier, the severity of the stroke determines the damage to the brain and hence the deficits one may have to overcome. A worker may therefore be required to change duties depending on their impairments. Therefore, stroke survivors need to be given care quickly and collaboratively in a manner that allows them to undertake tasks adequately and safely. Stroke survivors can still undertake safety-sensitive tasks, but under the observation of an occupational therapist. The occupational therapist can evaluate the safety requirements hazards, risks, and exposures the patients may be putting themselves or other people in if they have a stroke-related problem. In reality, a stroke survivor can't walk out of a clinic after therapy and then be driving an oil rig across town. Employers also need to support stroke survivors back to work. Stroke survivors are encouraged to make constant visits to their place of work before their return so as to decrease the anxiety and apprehension they or the employer may have. With the help of an occupational health, the return to work can be made as gradual as possible. (Phased return is available on MED 3 Certificates with adjustments, if required.)

In conclusion, it is possible to fully return to work after a stroke. It may take three to eight or even more months, depending on the severity of the stroke, rate of recovery, and the work one is going back to, but it is possible with the right care. It is actually heartening to both clinicians and family members to have a stroke patient go back to work. Even then, the patient should be assessed continually for invisible impairments.

My Return to Work

After my brain haemorrhage and brain surgery, I felt very depressed and exhausted. As a result, mentally I was in a very bad place. Not only did I have brain surgery, but there was a rare underlying condition I had never researched.

I couldn't work as a GP initially because I was tired all the time. Even though I could empathise with my patients, I was not ready for a GP role. Instead I worked with the local council on the exercise referral scheme. I also did some care work. It was very tiring doing visits thirty minutes to one hour, preparing lunches, and getting the elderly ready for the day.

Being a care giver was natural and rewarding for me. I could take histories from clients, call the doctors, and arrange home visits. Great, if I wasn't so tired.

I finally decided to do a job that consisted of repetitive actions. I went to work in a food manufacturing company. Well, I was rubbish at standing in a production line. I was always behind, despite rotation to different chores, but even with a medical degree, I could not work for six hours with thirty-five-minute breaks. I was suffering from repetitive sprain injury from piping chocolate for one hour. The products were great, but I was not suited to this type of work. I watched my colleagues perform really well. The EU citizens I worked with were very talented in this work and managed to fill most of the posts as managers and section leaders. I am not sure what is going to happen to all talented workers from EU countries after Brexit.

References

Watson S. (2019) Getting Back to Work after a Stroke: Only half of stroke survivors make it back into the workforce, study shows. Retrieved on June 24, 2019 from https://www.webmd.com/stroke/news/20080327/getting-back-to-work-after-a-stroke#1

Westerlind, E., Persson, H. C., & Sunnerhagen, K. S. (2017). Return to Work after a Stroke in Working Age Persons; A Six-Year Follow Up. PloS one, 12(1), e0169759. doi:10.1371/journal.pone.0169759. Retrieved on June 24, 2019 from https://www.ncbi.nlm.nih.gov/pmc/articles/PMC5218734/

Castaneda R. (2018) 9 Reasons You Should Return to Work After a Stroke. Retrieved on June 24, 2019 from https://health.usnews.com/health-care/patient-advice/slideshows/9-reasons-you-should-return-to-work-after-a-stroke

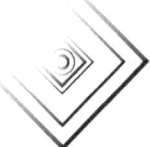

PAIN AFTER STROKE

CENTRAL POST-STROKE PAIN (CPSP) AND NEUROPATHIC PAIN

Stroke survivors are full of fear and anxiety that it may happen again, especially when they feel or experience pain in their body. Different people feel pain differently; one of the first steps in dealing with pain is to know or understand the cause of the pain.

Pain after stroke is actually a very common symptom which can manifest immediately, or in weeks, or even months or years after the stroke event. Although pain after stroke is commonly reported, it is usually managed incompletely, especially due its esoteric nature and the fact that post-stroke pain has not been covered much in recent stroke management discussions. Pain after stroke is usually not understood properly by practitioners. Actually it is easily overlooked because it has variable characteristics. It may occur together with comorbid medical problems, and the patient may not express this affliction due to impairments in communication and cognition. Recent studies report that neuropathic pain is the most common and frequent type of pain-after stroke, and since such pain syndromes are unique to individual patients, it may not be managed sufficiently. This leads to the need to delineate it based on the pathophysiology

Central Post-Stroke Pain (CPSP)

Neuropathic pain is one of the major symptoms affecting stroke survivors. The term *central post-stroke pain* does not refer to the actual pain but describes the symptoms of pain that arise after a stroke. As is the case with all strokes, the character of the deficit is dictated by the location of the damage and the neurologic function of the affected structure. In neuropathic pain, the lesion affects some part of the central pain pathways, causing a painful sensation without stimulating the peripheral pain receptors. Since the pain-processing pathways of the brain cannot sense the pain, the brain, which is used to receiving normal sensory inputs, goes ahead and produces the painful sensation itself.

Neuropathic pain is quite difficult to characterise because patients can subjectively describe it in a myriad of ways. Stroke survivors suffering from neuropathic pain may present with a range of ailments from an aching, dull sharp to throbbing, stabbing, burning, or shooting pain. Central post-stroke pain may also feel like a numbness of prickling on the skin. In most cases, the pain is felt on the side of the body that was affected by the stroke. Also, neuropathic pain tends to worsen if the affected part is placed in water or if the patient si touched or moved. Neuropathic pain can be quite uncomfortable and can potentially impact the recovery process. It means that one will experience different types of pain due to CPSP. The onset of neuropathic pain is also variable with the most common cases beginning from one to three months after the stroke. Most patients, however, report developing CPSP symptoms by the fifth to sixth month after stroke. CPSP can also begin weeks and even years after stroke. There is no precise timeline for the onset.

The duration of neuropathic pain tends to last for a longer time—days, weeks, and even much longer. Such chronic pain tends to continue, even when the affected part of the brain has healed.

Anatomical Association of Neuropathic Pain

A brief history about neuropathic pain shows that it dates back in 1906 when Dejerine and Roussy first described it using the phrase *'syndrome thalamique,'* meaning thalamic syndrome. They described it as an intolerable pain in the hemiplegic side of patients who were found to have survived strokes affecting the thalamus. As such, for many years, the thalamus seemed the most accepted source of neuropathic pain, which was even referred to as Dejerine-Roussy syndrome. However, more recent studies and reports show that the thalamus happens to be one of the brain structures that are implicated in CPSP. It is now clear that neuropathic pain occurs in patients whose lesion, due to stroke, affects any of the neural tracts that are responsible for transmitting pain as they reach the entire central nervous system. One such tract is the spinothalamic tract.

The spinothalamic tract has been studied widely in association to neuropathic pain. This tract transmits particular senses of pain, deep touch, and temperature from the body. Its general course begins at the lateral part of the spinal cord via the lateral pons and medulla, then through the ventral posterolateral nucleus of the thalamus, and terminates at the post-central gyrus (Treister et al. 2017). Any injury or lesion to a part in this path of the tract can potentially cause neuropathic pain. However, some parts like the thalamus tend to be associated with central pain syndrome than others.

The thalamus happens to be one of the most studied and documented neural structures in relation to neuropathic pain. This explains why neuropathic pain was originally known as thalamic pain. More studies show CPSP patients usually have lesions in their ventral posteromedial (VPM) and the posterolateral nucleus (VPL) of the thalamus. A more recent study that incorporated digital radiographic atlases and MRI imaging in patients who had survived thalamic stroke and had or lacked neuropathic pain showed that patients with neuropathic pain had lesions that largely involved the VPL and VPM nucleus (Brunecker et al. 2012). Another study has also showed that if the thalamic lesion involves the section where the ventral posterior nucleus meets the pulvinar, then the patient is more than eighty times more likely to suffer CPSP compared to other thalamic lesions. As such, the thalamus is a high-risk area for neuropathic pain, implying that potential treatments against neuropathic pain should focus on such avenues of research (Treister et al. 2017).

The cerebral cortex also has areas which are associated with neuropathic pain while others are not. In a study of twenty-four patients, it was found that an ischemic injury to the insular and operculum cortex was associated with the development of CPSP.

Pathophysiology of Neuropathic Pain

It is not yet clear which pathophysiology does neuropathic pain arise with after stroke. There are, however, factors which researchers have identified as important indicators for the development of neuropathic pain. These include stroke severity, a history of depression, smoking, and stroke at a young age. Post-operative pain following a craniotomy can last for years. One of the most widely accepted theories uses disinhibition to explain neuropathic pain. In simple words, lesions or injuries to the brain's sensory pathways cause a compensatory overactivation of the thalamus, thus resulting in a spontaneous allodynia—pain produced by an unpainful stimulus (Treister et al. 2017).

Treatment of Neuropathic Pain

Neuropathic pain cannot be treated by using ordinary painkillers. Ordinary prescriptions for pain, like ibuprofen and paracetamol, have proven unhelpful in alleviating neuropathic pain. There are, however, a variety of psychoactive and *neuromodulating medications* which are useful to treating CPSP. In addition, neuropathic pain can be treated using non-pharmacologic measures.

Anticonvulsants are antiepileptic drugs and many of them have been used to treat neuropathic pain. The most popular choice includes calcium channel modulators like *gabapentin* and *pregabalin*. According to a placebo-controlled 2019 study, pregabalin may not reduce the pain significantly but it improves the patients' sleep, anxiety, and other qualities of life. It should also be noted that pregabalin has adverse side effects like dizziness, oedema, somnolence, and weight gain. Another study showed a significant long-term efficacy in using pregabalin whereby the subjective pain in patient who respond to the drug improves significantly over a fifty-two-week period. The study also reported a good tolerability of the pregabalin treatment despite its high incidence of side effects. As a result, gabapentin is usually the first line of treatment for treating neuropathic pain because it has a flexible dosage and is relatively affordable (Treister et al. 2017).

Sodium channel blockers are other anticonvulsants used to treat pain. Carbamazepine is one such drug currently considered as the second line treatment for neuropathic pain. It is, however, less efficacious due to its higher incidence of adverse effects like aplastic anaemia and Stevens-Johnson syndrome. Despite its effects and interaction with other medications, carbamazepine is still used because of its historical success in treating neuropathic pain.

Other medications include antidepressants like *amitriptyline*. This tricyclic antidepressant was shown to be significantly effective in treating neuropathic pain back in 1989. This medication was shown to be both safe and effective at a daily dosage of seventy-five milligrams. The drug has some side effects like constipation, dry mouth, orthostatic hypertension, and urinary retention; however, is should be considered that this particular drug lowers the seizure threshold (Leojon and Boivie 1989).

Other drugs, like serotonin reuptake inhibitors and corticosteroids, are potential treatments for pain. Since most of the medications mentioned above can cause severe and sometimes dangerous side effects, the patient suffering from neuropathic pain should have the physician assess the best medication the patient can tolerate based on pain severity, age, and other comorbidities to arrive at a safe regimen for treatment and max adherence to medication (Treister et al. 2017).

Non-pharmacologic treatments can be called for if the medication is not tolerable. Deep brain stimulation is one very promising treatment. This treatment is particularly necessary for severe neuropathic pain, the kind that does not get better with medication. The procedure involves implanting a medical device into the brain and sending electric signals via electrodes placed in the brain to the target neural structure. This method is effective in treating chronic pain syndromes and offers relief in various degrees. Neuropathic pain is a complex and complicated phenomenon, but it is treatable and manageable in manner that makes life more normal and satisfactory.

My Experience of Pain after Stroke and Brain Surgery

I was unfortunate to have pain from my subarachnoid haemorrhage, cardiodynia, due to occlusion of my internal carotid arteries and ongoing discomfort at my craniotomy site. During craniotomy surgery, specialised instruments are used to remove a bone flap. It can take one to four weeks or even a few years to adjust to the altered sensation at the craniotomy site.

I found a temperature change and windy days made my craniotomy pain worse. On occasion, a severe pain can interrupt my daily routine. The only medication I found helpful was amitriptyline in doses of fifty milligrams. This can make you feel drowsy. It is suggested to take last thing at night, and it may help with sleep and depression. I was very familiar with prescribing amitriptyline as a GP. Many of my patients referred to it as the blue tablet.

I didn't get on with other anticonvulsant drugs used in management of chronic pain like gabapentin or pregabalin. Weight gain was a side effect that concerned me, and feeling lightheaded, and I was trying to avoid dependence on these drugs.

Amitriptyline has been available to prescribe for neuropathic pain for a very long time. I find it very useful to help me sleep. I am less anxious and have reduced pain from my scar.

I usually wear a woollen hat to make my scar feel more comfortable.

The trouble with a stroke with no visible symptoms is everyone just assumes you are fine, but in fact, most days are a struggle.

Reference Krause T, Brunecker P, Pittl S, et al. Thalamic sensory strokes with and without pain:
differences in psychiatry. 2012 Aug; 83(8):776–784. Retrieved on 9 July 2019 from https://www.ncbi.nlm.nih.gov/pubmed/22696587

Leijon, G., and Boivie, J. (1989). Central post-stroke pain—a controlled trial of amitriptyline and carbamazepine. Pain, 36(1), 27-36. Retrieved on 9 July, 2019 from https://www.sciencedirect.com/science/article/pii/0304395989901085

Sprenger, T., Seifert, C. L., Valet, M., Andreou, A. P., Foerschler, A., Zimmer, C. and Chakravarty, M. M. (2012). Assessing the risk of central post-stroke pain of thalamic origin by lesion mapping. Brain, 135(8), 2536-2545. Retrieved on 9 July, 2019 from https://academic.oup.com/brain/article-abstract/135/8/2536/305095

Treister, A. K., Hatch, M. N., Cramer, S. C., and Chang, E. Y. (2017). Demystifying poststroke pain: from etiology to treatment. PMandR, 9(1), 63-75. Retrieved on 9 July 2019 from https://www.sciencedirect.com/science/article/pii/S1934148216301824

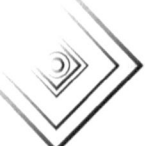

Exercise after Stroke

Exercising is good for everyone's health. The same applies for stroke survivors. Of course, the obvious understanding is that for stroke survivors, their mobility may be limited or restricted. There are numerous barriers to a stroke survivor's physical activity. Some of them include fatigue, depression, and even disability. However, it is still possible to get some form of exercise, provided they start slowly as they find a way around the physical barriers. Physical exercise is extremely important because it not only improves the recovery process but also prevents and reduces the risk of having another stroke. It is, however, unfortunate that, despite the many health benefits of exercise to stroke survivors, not very many healthcare professionals will prescribe it as form of therapy. In addition, most stroke survivors lack the knowledge support and tools needed for them to begin an exercise programme. This section hopes to change all that.

Physical activity by definition is the human movement caused by actions of the skeletal muscles and substantially increasing the energy expenditure. Physical exercise is a key subset under physical activity. It generally means having physical activities that are planned, structured, and performed deliberately and in a repetitive manner with the intention to improve one's physical fitness (Saunders et al. 2014). There are several indicators of physical fitness. They include muscle strength, cardiorespiratory fitness, and muscle power, all of which determine one's capacity to not only perform but also tolerate physical activity. Physical fitness becomes severely impaired after a stroke; a stroke survivor's cardiorespiratory fitness peak reduces to 50 per cent less than that of a healthy person of the same sex and age. There are also impairments in muscle power and muscle strength as well as in bilateral limb weakness, which are a clear indication of physical inactivity.

Physical inactivity or the lack of exercise is a risk factor for stroke. According to the Stroke Foundation, exercising reduces the risk of having a transient ischaemic attack or stroke by more than 25 per cent when done moderately for half an hour every day (Mcilroy 2017). Finding a sustainable exercise plan should therefore be an important part of the recovery process for every stroke survivor because it prevents a stroke from recurring.

Potential Benefits of Exercise after Stroke

Even for healthy people, exercise is highly recommended because it has positive contributions to the health, fitness, and functioning of all people in the general population. Exercise provides for one's mental and physical health, lowering cholesterol levels and blood pressure. It also helps reduce the risk of heart problems like type 2 diabetes, helps reduce depression and anxiety levels, and helps lose weight and maintain a healthy weight. In addition, exercise increases muscle flexibility and strength and is thus an added advantage for stroke survivors with motor function impairments. Exercise improves one's self-esteem and increases one's energy levels. For stroke survivors with sleep problems, exercise helps one sleep better. There are also certain fitness impairments which are common with functional limitations after stroke. Such limitations like walking can be casual, whereby the fitness impairments exacerbate or cause disability. Increasing physical exercise after stroke can therefore improve one's fitness as well as improve functional problems after stroke (Mcilroy 2017).

Current research evidence on exercise after stroke shows that exercise interventions are beneficial in addressing arm function, cognition, gait, and balance. Other potential benefits include confidence and fatigue. One has to approach exercise after stroke with the understanding that post-stroke disability is a complex phenomenon usually because the resulting damage due to the stroke as well as what goes on during the recovery process is not quite clear. For example, fatigue is one of the common and damaging symptoms after stroke. The causes of this kind of fatigue are not certain, but it is likely due to a combination of physiological and psychological mechanisms. Since after stroke one's physical fitness reduces greatly, the effort needed to carry out any physical activity becomes greater and more fatiguing. This is primarily why stroke survivors are advised to avoid or reduce their physical activity, but post-stroke fatigue doesn't get better with rest or inactivity. Several trials have shown that post-stroke fatigue reduces more when stroke survivors undergo cognitive therapy together with exercise intervention (Saunders et al. 2014).

Researches with regards to exercise have led to the development of exercise programmes tailored to the needs and specifications of stroke survivors. There are many choices of exercise, but the best choice will depend on one's interests and physical abilities as well as what one can find locally. One can opt to either exercise on one's own or join an exercise group or club. Some common exercise choices include walking, jogging, cycling, and swimming. One can even use an exercise computer programme to exercise at home. However, before getting active, one should consult one's GP, especially if it's the first time to exercise. This precaution is necessary because some medications can have side effects that will limit the choice of exercise. The Stroke Association in the United Kingdom recommends the aerobic exercise programme which significantly boosts stroke recovery (Saunders et al. 2014).

Aerobics and Strokeability

Aerobics is a key feature of Woking Strokeability, which is group programme providing aerobics together with aqua exercises, particularly for survivors of stroke or any similar disability. Strokeability is offered by professionals who understand the needs of stroke survivors with regards to physical activity limitations. Cardio exercise or aerobics is a planned and routine type of exercise where the body's oxygen is used to meet the body's energy demands. Good examples include biking, hiking, running, dancing, swimming, and any other activity whereby the breathing and heart rate increases at a sustainable rate. These activities do not allow one to run out of breath quickly. Aerobics aids in conditioning and strengthening muscles of the heart and those associated with respiration. As a result, the heart improves in pumping efficiency, blood pressure reduces, and the exercise generally facilitates air flow into and out of the lungs. Aerobic exercise should be this part of a stroke survivor's routine; it provides significant improvements in cognitive deficits for stroke survivors (Stroke Association 2019).

Stroke survivors, particularly those with mobility deficits, may avoid exercises or even lack knowledge on how to begin and maintain a routine. This is risky because they may start a dangerous cycle of not being physically active and thus their muscle weakness gets worse. As a result, one should first be screened by one's doctor or general practitioner, be cleared, and then begin aerobics exercise—the earlier the better after the stroke. The screening is important because it helps the doctor set exercise goals and identify medical conditions requiring specific accommodation during aerobics exercise. For example, it is possible to engage fully in aerobics while sitting. The screening also helps come up with an exercise routine or programme that meets one's needs and capabilities. Strokeability programmes usually involve therapists to help in supervising and monitoring the aerobics exercises, but eventually the goal as a stroke survivor is to exercise independently (Mcilroy 2017).

At first it may be possible to reach the recommended thirty minutes of moderate aerobic exercise for five days every week, but any amount is better than nothing. One should work with one's GP to set realistic goals. In case the routine causes any discomfort or pain or worsens prevailing symptoms, one should stop the exercise immediately and contact one's healthcare provider and therapist to modify the exercise and make it more sustainable (Saunders et al. 2014).

In conclusion, everyone needs some kind of motivation to exercise, and usually the first step of getting started is the most difficult. This can be particularly harder for a stroke survivor because one can't enjoy participating in activities one did before the stroke. But as hard as it may be, the realisation that exercise is an important part of the rehabilitation and recovery from stroke should get one started. Once the benefits start manifesting, it won't be easy to stop exercising.

My Stroke and Exercise

I am an odd one really because when I recommenced running after my brain operation, I was determined and resilient and still very competitive to secure two more five-kilometre, open-race trophies.

To help improve my post-stroke fitness, I did a fitness course. I did a level 3 diploma in exercise referral, which taught me to exercise safely and monitor my body afterwards. Yes, there are times when I run in wild countryside and think, *Oh dear. There is no signal here. The ambulance will say they can't find me if I collapse.* It is important to alert your loved ones if you go on a walk in an isolated area. Not that they will come, but they might send help if needed.

I also wear a medical bracelet with my details and condition to allow an ambulance to start resuscitation in the event of a collapse/further stroke. I still push myself. My donor graft has allowed me to do so as it has 'matured' with age.

References

Mcilroy, W. (2017) 'Exercise and Stroke Recovery', pp. 1–8. Retrieved from https://www.stroke.org.uk/sites/default/files/exercise_and_stroke.pdf

Stroke Association (2019) Woking Strokeability. Retrieved from https://www.stroke.org.uk/finding-support/woking-strokeability

Saunders, D. H., Greig, C. A., & Mead, G. E. (2014). Physical activity and exercise after stroke: review of multiple meaningful benefits. Stroke, 45(12), 3742-3747. Retrieved from https://www.ahajournals.org/doi/full/10.1161/strokeaha.114.004311

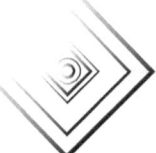

ALCOHOL AND BRAIN INJURY

This section is rather interesting. It is not about how or whether alcohol causes brain injury. It is about how people with some type of brain injury deal with alcohol consumption. It is important to mention that a significant percentage of people with traumatic brain injury have a history of drinking and alcohol abuse.

Alcohol use and traumatic brain injury are closely related. Staying away from alcohol is strongly recommended after brain injury.

The general observation has been that having alcohol after brain injury, one's brain is more sensitive to alcohol. Brain injury can feel overwhelming even on a mild serving of alcohol. Most people with brain injuries have reported that their brains tend to feel more sensitive to alcohol. The relationship between brain injury and alcohol is complex. Although the exact causes are not very clear, this chapter can give more insight.

A stroke happens when blood supply to the brain is cut off. Other types of brain injury include a car crash which causes the brain to bounce around the skull, causing tears and bruises called contusions and even haemorrhage, which is invisible bleeding of the brain. Any trauma that penetrates the skull can reach the brain and potentially cause a brain injury. So alcohol can become problematic for an injured brain (Headway 2018).

Alcohol is one of the most popular drinks. It is a drug that is very common in recreational and social activities. Its general effect is making you feel relaxed, letting you blow the steam off and enjoy life after a long day's work.

Alcohol can negatively affect several skills like memory, information processing, attention, mobility, and balance, etc.—even in a perfectly healthy person who has *not* had a brain injury (Headway 2018). It therefore makes sense why a person with a brain injury can feel overwhelmed by all the resulting reactions since *even without alcohol, brain injury alone can* cause all the mentioned side effects of alcohol. This scenario does not refer to alcohol misuse, which is still a largely undocumented problem among people who have survived a traumatic brain injury. Instead, it refers to a mild to moderate consumption of alcohol—one or two drinks per day. Of course, there are studies that suggest that taking such moderate alcohol consumptions has some positive health benefits, including even lowering the risk of stroke, but in reality, alcohol does not auger well with any brain injury.

The Pathophysiology of Alcohol and the Brain

Alcohol mainly affects the brain's prefrontal cortex, the part responsible for processing information, making decisions, and monitoring behaviour. What actually happens when a person who has had a brain injury takes alcohol is quite simple. Because of the brain injury, the brain or the person's tolerance to alcohol reduces. The stroke or brain injury survivor feels more sensitive to alcohol because the brain cannot handle alcohol the same way it did before the injury (Headway 2018). This can lead to a stroke survivor becoming unsure of what precise amount of alcohol is too much or safe—or even whether they should be taking alcohol in the first place. The increased sensitivity or the low tolerance to alcohol is the brain's way of saying things are not as they used to be. The brain has to embark on numerous and unimaginable tasks of self-repair, reconnecting and rewiring damaged brain cells, neural functions, and even regenerating new brain cells and neural paths through neurogenesis (Bjorklund and Lindvall 2000). Alcohol tends to hinder this crucial part of the recovery process.

Research shows that taking alcohol after a brain injury increases the risk of getting another brain injury. Worst of all, alcohol slows down and can even stop the recovery process of the brain (Frank et al. 2010). The risk of developing seizures increases with alcohol consumption after brain injury. In this case, the alcohol lowers the seizure threshold or can just trigger seizures. Survivors who do not take alcohol are thus at a lesser risk of having seizures. The negative effects of a brain injury are similar to those of alcohol because both affect the mental ability. With alcohol, these effects actually become magnified and the resulting effects tend to last longer even after one stops drinking. If, for example, the survivor takes some antidepressants, it is advisable to stay away from any level of alcohol. Using alcohol causes and worsens depression, which is a common effect especially during the first year after a traumatic brain injury. Despite the temporally relaxing effect it has, alcohol worsens depression and causes or exacerbates mood disorders. *Alcohol will interfere with most medications prescribed after a brain injury.*

Alcohol is dangerous after a brain injury, and since it makes some prescriptions less effective, it causes more severe side effects. It can lead to an overdose and even death. This applies to a range of drugs including painkillers and anti-anxiety medications (Frank et al. 2010).

These facts emphasise the fact that no amount of alcohol is ever safe after a traumatic brain injury. The brain's recovery process takes longer than one can imagine, and the improvements can become noticeable many years after the injury. Avoiding alcohol is one of the best ways to give the brain the best chance of improvement. Many brain injury survivors have given up drinking during their first year after the stroke or brain injury. That is probably because during that period they were in a rehabilitation centre or a setting where they could not access alcohol or get back to their previous drinking habits

(Headway 2018). Such individuals are at a higher risk of drinking alcohol again, especially when they are back to their home setting. Taking alcohol might actually seem like their way of adjusting to life after the injury, but even if they become occasional drinkers, the alcohol does more harm and no good to their recovery.

Brain injuries differ in terms of severity and the brain function or part that is affected. A few stroke survivors, who probably lack insight, drink moderately, regularly, or even heavily and depend on alcohol to cope. After brain injury, drink responsibly. But the best insight is to stay away from consuming alcohol after a brain injury.

My Experience with Alcohol

I found myself initially feeling relaxed and less anxious after ingesting alcohol. After one year of my operation, I noticed that a smaller amount of alcohol was making me more aggressive and very confused. This was worse after I took my painkillers for headaches and pain at the site of the scar.

My example of the worst effect of alcohol was being arrested for a disturbance in a pub and common assault. I cannot remember the event, but waking up in custody was a wake-up call. I admitted myself into an alcohol rehabilitation unit for four weeks because I had to stop any volume of alcohol.

The experience was useful for me because for the first time I had to confront my personal demons. There was no longer an escape. I had to get to the root cause of unhappiness through open group discussions and assignments. It offered counselling and relaxation methods and offered me support after rehabilitation.

References

Björklund, A., & Lindvall, O. (2000). Neurobiology: self-repair in the brain. *Nature, 405*(6789), 892. Retrieved on July 20, 2019 from https://www.nature.com/articles/35016175

Frank, R. G., Rosenthal, M., & Caplan, B. (2010). *Handbook of rehabilitation psychology*. American Psychological Association. Retrieved on July 20, 2019 from https://psycnet.apa.org/record/2009-19679-000

Headway (2018). Alcohol after brain injury. *The Brain Injury Association*. Factsheet. Retrieved on July 20, 2019 from https://www.headway.org.uk/media/5800/alcohol-after-brain-injury-factsheet.pdf

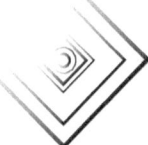

PSYCHOTHERAPY AFTER STROKE

Psychotherapy includes treatment plans intended for a broad range of mental illnesses. It is also known as talk therapy or talk treatment. Instead of using medication, it entails talking with a therapist. Psychotherapy can be used for people with emotional difficulties, mood challenges, mental health problems, or psychiatric disorders. It can similarly be used as an aid in controlling or eliminating troubling symptoms that may hinder one from functioning better or improving one's healing and well-being.

Stroke survivors depict a myriad of mental conditions which can be successfully treated using psychotherapy. Theoretically, the same principal treatments for depression in the general population should work in stroke patients. However, since stroke survivors differ from the general population in terms of the severity and extent of their mental condition, psychotherapy may serve them differently.

In stroke survivors, the most common symptom is depression. A stroke survivor has a 25 per cent to 70 per cent of developing depression. Most research studies suggest approximately a 30 per cent frequency rate of having depression after stroke (APA 2018). The most consistent findings indicate that most stroke survivors experience low moods which require medical and psychological intervention. As mentioned in an earlier chapter, depression is caused by a myriad of biochemical changes which take place within the brain in the event of a brain injury. One of the possible outcomes after a brain injury is that the patient becomes unable to experience positive emotions. This marks the onset of depression because it starts a chain reaction of emotional problems and mood challenges like anxiety, irritability, hopelessness, fatigue, lack of concentration, insomnia, loss of appetite and even suicidal thoughts (American Stroke Association 2018).

Psychological therapies have a very high efficacy in treating people with anxiety (Stroke Foundation 2018). There is, however, a scarcity of studies that employ psychological intervention in treating depression in stroke patients. Talk therapy is usually considered as a treatment for depression in stroke patients by combining it with medication, thus improving the patient's success rate.

There are at least seven types of psychotherapy, and each one addresses a particular aspect or condition in a patient. In reality, the type of therapy choice will depend on the type of mental illness as well as the patient's preference. The patient's preference is crucial because talk therapy may prove impossible if the patient cannot talk or express their condition by communicating with the therapist. It is also possible for the therapist to combine various types of psychotherapy to meet the needs of the patient and achieve the best results. Psychotherapy involves the use of scientifically valid methods to help the patient adopt more effective and healthier habits. In reality and in practice, anyone, including a stroke survivor, can benefit from psychotherapy. There have been several inconclusive studies which either used a limited or biased sample size and arrived at the conclusion that psychotherapy is not effective in treating depression after stroke. Such studies recommend for further randomised studies (Lincoln and Flannaghan 2003).

Cognitive Behavioural Therapy (CBT)

Cognitive behavioural therapy is an approach used by therapists to help stroke patients identify and eliminate behaviours or thinking patterns that are ineffective or harmful to their recovery process. CBT helps patients replace such thoughts and behaviour with more functional behaviours and accurate, positive thoughts. CBT is so far the most effective approach for treating depression in elderly patients as well as the general population. Despite the scarcity of studies, there are numerous indications that CBT is as successful in treating depression among stroke patients. One report (Lincoln and Flannaghan 2003) studied nineteen stroke patients by taking them through a ten-session, four-week baseline CBT period. The study revealed that CBT has a tendency of improving the mood among stroke patients. Only four out of the nineteen patients reported significant mood improvement after CBT. As such, the conclusion was that CBT was effective in some stroke patients (Lincoln and Flannaghan 2003).

Interpersonal Therapy IPT

Interpersonal therapy is a short-term psychotherapy approach. It involves the therapist helping the patient understand certain interpersonal issues that might be troubling them, such as a change in work or social roles and problems relating with other people. Such interpersonal issues are common symptoms among stroke survivors. IPT is an effective approach in teaching stroke patients healthier ways of improving their communication, expressing their emotions, and how they can relate to others. IPT is used as a treatment for depression.

Dialectical Therapy

Psychodynamic therapy is a form of CBT that is aimed at regulating emotions. It is mostly employed in treating patients who exhibit eating disorders, PTSD, borderline personality disorders, and chronic suicidal thoughts. Dialectical therapy works by teaching the patients new skills which help them take personal responsibility and change their disruptive or unhealthy behaviour. Dialectical behavioural therapy can be conducted in either group or individual therapy sessions.

Supportive Therapy

Supportive therapy is an approach through which the therapist guides and encourages the patients to acquire psychological resources by themselves. This involves guiding and helping them build their self-esteem, strengthen their coping mechanisms, reduce anxiety, and even improve their communities and social functioning. Through the help of supportive therapy, patients can deal with their mental health issues which affect a huge part of their lives.

The above types of psychotherapy address mental and behavioural conditions which also affect stroke patients. As such, these psychotherapy approaches can be used to treat particular conditions in patients after stroke. Previous researches have established that depression is a prevalent condition among stroke patients. It is capable of hindering, slowing, or compromising the effectiveness of pharmaceutical treatment and physical therapy. A stroke patient with depression and anxiety can, for example, have difficulty exercising at home, staying motivated and focused, or even taking medication as prescribed.

Stroke is a serious, overwhelming, and life-changing event. It affects how people feel about themselves and how they relate with their friends and family. It also affects one's role in work, family, and finances and thus can cause stress, anxiety, and sadness. There is an established connection between stroke anxiety and depression (APA 2019). Suffering a stroke also results in personality, emotional, and mood disorders. These conditions can be overwhelming to stroke survivors, considering that they had just suffered brain damage. As such, the use of psychotherapeutic approaches in the treatment of stroke is a highly recommended method to address the patients' psychological needs and help them through the challenges of recovering.

There have been myths and stigma associated with seeking psychotherapeutic intervention. However, such baseless reasons should no longer deter anyone from seeking help. Depression after stroke is treatable, and it is important to note that the success of psychotherapy relies on the creation and maintenance of a trusting relationship between the patient and the therapist (APA 2019). Currently, getting help through psychotherapy is a sign of resourcefulness since taking care of one's mental health is a proven way to ensure good physical health. This is according to the mind-body connection which emphasises that emotional problems can manifest physically while physical illness can manifest as emotional issues. Stroke survivors have emotional issues which may affect their physical health. Thus, they deserve the best chance to improve their physical and mental life during the recovery stage.

My Experience with Psychotherapy

Four years after my stroke, I began to realise the enormity of what had happened to me. Following my police arrest in September 2016 for assault, I became scared for my own safety and became a vulnerable adult.

My forensic history and associated minor behavioural changes like overspending without concern for the future led me see various neuropsychiatrists/neuropsychologists for neuro rehab. Being a doctor, my executive functioning played a significant part in my future career choices. I underwent baseline neuropsychological assessments, and this had to be repeated at intervals to detect any deterioration in my cognition.

The loss of work as a GP, marital disharmony and subsequent divorce, and building a more stable relationship with my daughter and the rest of my family significantly affected my mood. I became severely depressed with poor appetite and weight loss of twenty kilograms. I was tearful and took an overdose on a few occasions. I was not coping with the burden I had become to others. I used running as an anchor for theses hard periods. The doctor prescribed antidepressants and anti-anxiolytic medication. These helped in managing the more physical symptoms like insomnia and loss of appetite.

What worked for me was talking therapy. It is not in my culture to share your dirty laundry with others. I attended weekly appointments for twelve weeks to address the management of different behaviours and positive thoughts using cognitive behavioural therapies. I looked forward to each session. I was free to talk, cry, and be honest with myself at how it was all going to take a very long time.

Some cognitive behavioural therapy waiting lists can be up to eighteen months. It is worth getting a book on self-help CBT. It will require patience and offer you some understanding of what you have been through.

My psychiatric ICD diagnosis includes the following:

- impulsive disorder
- cognitive impairment
- organic personality change
- recurrent depressive disorder

All are made worse by the consumption of even a small amount of alcohol.

It is very important to attend your neuropsychology appointments. Neuropsychologists are trained to understand the cognitive, emotional, and behavioural effects in a wide range of brain conditions. The neuropsychology services are limited, so expect a waiting list.

References

American Psychological Association (APA) (2019). Understanding psychotherapy and how it works. Retrieved on 26 August 2019 from: https://www.apa.org/helpcenter/understanding-psychotherapy

American Stroke Association (2018). Depression and Stroke. Retrieved on 26 August 2019 from: https://www.stroke.org/en/about-stroke/effects-of-stroke/emotional-effects-of-stroke/depression-and-stroke

Lincoln, & Flannaghan. (2003). Cognitive Behavioral Psychotherapy for Depression Following Stroke | Stroke. Retrieved 26 August 2019, from https://www.ahajournals.org/doi/full/10.1161/01.STR.0000044167.44670.55

WebMD (2011) Motivational Therapy Helps Treat Stroke Patients. Retrieved on 26 August 2019 from: https://www.webmd.com/stroke/news/20110623/motivational-therapy-helps-treat-stroke-patients#2

www.ingramcontent.com/pod-product-compliance
Lightning Source LLC
Chambersburg PA
CBHW031536210526
45464CB00003B/1038